FULLY FIT IN 60 MINUTES A WEEK

The Complete Shape-Up Programme for Women

by

Susanne O'Sullivan

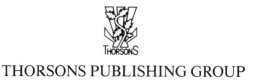

THORSONS PUBLISHING GROUP

First published in the United Kingdom April 1984

Original American edition published by
Tribeca Communications, Inc., New York

18   20   19

British Library Cataloguing in Publication Data

O'Sullivan, Susanne
Fully fit in 60 minutes a week: the
complete shape-up programme for women.
1. Physical fitness for women
I. Title
613.7'045   RA781

ISBN 0-7225-1848-X

*Published by Thorsons Publishers Limited,
Wellingborough, Northamptonshire, NN8 2RQ, England.*

Printed in Great Britain by Woolnough Bookbinding,
Irthlingborough, Northamptonshire

About the Author

Susanne O'Sullivan is a life-long disciple of fitness and physical activity. A gymnast and dancer since age six, she is an avid long-distance runner and has developed many programs for muscular strength, flexibility, endurance, and cardiovascular fitness.

Acknowledgements

Thank you to Bill Laznovsky and Todd Estabrook for their able assistance in designing the exercise programs; Doris Tucker for her accurate manuscript typing; Lisa Marsoli for her careful copyediting; Jim Parker for his exacting work behind the camera; and John Monteleone of Mountain Lion Books for tying up all the loose ends and producing this book on schedule.

Credits: Photography by James Whittier Parker of Gerard Photo, Hamilton Township, N.J. Produced by Mountain Lion Books, N.Y. City and Rocky Hill, N.J. Designed by Connie Kellner, Publishers TypeCenter, Morrisville, Pa. Jacket designed by Dilip Kane.

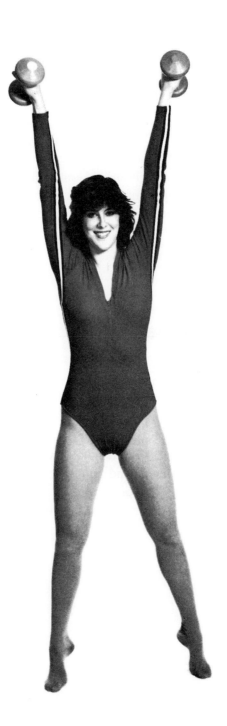

Table of Contents

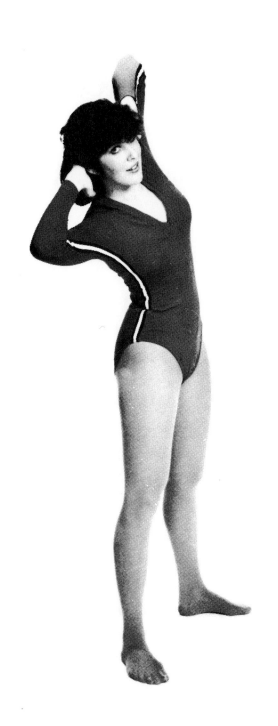

Introduction

Take a minute to give yourself a long hard look in the mirror. Chances are you're not really satisfied with what you see. You don't like to admit it, but those midnight snacks and junk food binges have finally caught up with you.

What to do?

You can cover up every mirror in the house *or* you can begin using this book to become physically fit in 60 minutes per week. The catch? Well, we're not selling starvation diets or miracle snake oil; few things in life come easy and exercise is no exception. But, by carefully following this book, within four to eight weeks we will give you a body you've never had before! But again, *you* must make the effort; with a sincere desire, dedication, and one hour a week of your time, *you can do it!*

Fully Fit In

60

Minutes a Week

is a series of basic muscular/skeletal exercises that, in conjunction with supplemental aerobic activity, represents a complete fitness plan that will give you:

- an improved, healthy posture
- a conditioned body with muscle tone
- reduced body fat and cellulite
- a shapely, active looking figure

- muscular endurance and stamina
- flexibility
- strength and vigor

This program deals specifically with the typical major trouble spots for women:

- double chins
- arm flab/cellulite
- tummies
- hips
- thighs
- breasts

This program will not only help you to physically look your best, but it will improve your mental outlook too. When you look good, you feel good.

By carefully following the format and *adhering to your schedule,* you will begin to see and feel tangible improvements after the first two weeks. Within six to eight weeks with self-discipline and 60 minutes a week, you *will* have the body of your dreams.

Before starting any new exercise program it is always best to have a medical checkup. This is a must if you have any serious medical conditions or if you are taking medication. Consult with your doctor before you begin.

Why be fit?

For millions of people, a normal day of largely sedentary work is an exhausting experience. It requires virtually 100% of their available energy, leaving them only enough to occasionally change the channel on their TV sets or fix themselves a nighttime snack. As a result, many people get far less out of life than they might if only they had more energy.

This need for more energy is one of the best answers to the question "Why be fit?" A person with a good degree of physical fitness will use only 60 to 70 percent of his or her energy capacity for routine daily activities. All the rest, some 30 to 40 percent, will be available for recreational and other activities.

But that's only the beginning. People who are physically fit are generally healthier. And when they do get sick, they usually recover faster. Often physically fit people are more attractive. They have less fat and more muscle and their skin may have that healthy glow that comes from regular exercise. Often too, a physically fit person is sharper mentally and able to do his or her work more efficiently.

Physical fitness also brings with it a certain pride and sense of well–being. And when your body and mind are functioning as they were meant to function, you simply feel better all over. What's more, by being physically fit you'll not only get more out of life, you'll also greatly improve your chances of living and enjoying life longer.

Unfortunately, since it's possible to exist without being physically fit, many people consider fitness a non-essential "extra" — something that would be nice to have if they could spare the time for it, but not one of life's true necessities. Or they see it as something that's fine for other people but not for them.

Nothing could be further from the truth. We live in a society where exercise is the exception, not the rule. And when the human body is not active, it inevitably degenerates. The muscles become weak and flabby, the joints begin to stiffen, and the lungs and heart become steadily less efficient. Or to put it another way, as far as your body's concerned, *if you don't use it, you lose it.*

Because of this, the choice is not between being fit and not being fit. It's between being fit and allowing our bodies to degenerate. Exercise and fitness are too important to be put off for lack of time. The programs in FULLY FIT IN 60 MINUTES A WEEK are designed to help you make maximum use of your limited exercise time — vigorous 20 minute workouts, three times a week.

The workouts on these pages specifically promote muscular strength and flexibility and when performed in conjunction with your choice of a cardiovascular activity — walking, jogging, swimming or biking on alternate days — they will leave you fully fit. Allow 30 to 60 days for maximum results.

Myths & Misconceptions

Over the years women interested in physical activity have been told discouraging myths about exercise and what it does to the female body.

So here, for the record, are the facts.

MYTH: *Women who exercise and/or lift weights end up with bulging muscles.*

FACT: The low level of testosterone (male hormone) present in women limits the development of bulky muscles found in males.

MYTH: *Exercise can actually reduce the size of your breasts.*

FACT: This is a classic example of conjecture based on ignorance. When you exercise frequently and intensively you burn calories, reducing the body's stores of fat. The result is a reduction in your overall weight. In no way can a general exercise program spot–reduce the breasts.

MYTH: *Vigorous exercise can harm a woman's reproductive organs.*

FACT: The truth of the matter is that the female reproductive organs, because they are internal and sheltered by the surrounding structure of the pelvis, are far less vulnerable to injury than the male organs. The uterus is actually the best protected organ in the female body, so it is highly unlikely that even very vigorous physical activity will harm a woman's reproductive organs.

MYTH: *Exercise can have an unfavorable long–term effect on childbirth.*

FACT: The great amount of research compiled on female athletes reveals conclusively that these women not only have normal pregnancies, but often experience easier childbirth with shorter delivery time. In fact, female Olympic athletes who become mothers have been found to have shorter second stages of labor compared to women in general, and this difference has been attributed to the athlete's superior muscle tone.

MYTH: *Exercise should cease with pregnancy.*

FACT: Contrary to this commonly held belief, appropriate exercise is in fact generally recommended by obstetricians who have realized that normal physical activity does not lead to spontaneous abortion. The more exercising you're used to, the more you can continue to do, up until the time you no longer feel comfortable exercising.

MYTH: *Exercise will permanently alter the menstrual cycle.*

FACT: For most female athletes training has no negative effects at all on the menstrual cycle. Occasionally, intense training required of the competitive athlete (such as the long–distance marathoner) can result in scant, infrequent, or even total cessation of periods (amenorrhea). Theories for these irregularities include a reaction to the stress of competition, and the decrease in body fat — common during training — leading to a change in estrogen metabolism. The effect however, has been shown to be only temporary and a decrease in the intensity of the physical activity will restore normal ovulatory function.

What is physical fitness?

Physical fitness promises a lot. Yet in spite of all the good things it produces, it isn't as hard to achieve as most people think. Unfortunately, the term has been so misused and misunderstood over the years that many people have the wrong idea of what it is and what it means. This misconception of what physical fitness is all about can sometimes prevent a person from ever achieving it.

For example, physical fitness definitely means more than not being sick, or merely being well. But it doesn't mean you have to be able to play four quarters of football or run the 26 miles for a marathon. Since the *average* level of fitness in this country is so low, being physically fit does mean being above average. But achieving a *normal* level of fitness is really all that's necessary. And to do that, you don't have to train eight hours a day like an Olympic champion.

Physical fitness is simply the ability to do your normal daily work with vigor and alertness, without undue fatigue, and with ample energy left over to enjoy leisure-time activities and to meet unforeseen emergencies. Normal physical fitness is thus a very reasonable goal that's well within the grasp of every user of FULLY FIT IN 60 MINUTES A WEEK.

What is Muscular Strength?

Muscular strength refers to the contraction power of the muscles. Each muscle in your body operates by contracting, often shortening itself by up to one half its total length. When you flex your arm, for example, one set of muscles contracts to pull it up. When you straighten it, the contractions of another set of muscles are involved.

Most people associate muscular strength with visible muscles like those found on professional body builders, and with the ability to lift heavy objects. That's fine as far as it goes, but it's important to be aware that muscular strength is also much, much more.

The human body has over 600 muscles, and almost every one of them is necessary for a normal, healthy life. Skeletal muscles, those attached to our bones, are essential to every move we make. Skeletal muscles are also responsible for holding our bodies in the proper posture so that internal organs can function efficiently. Other muscles are responsible for pulling air into our lungs, for moving food through the digestive tract, and for returning blood to the heart.

Muscles are truly marvelous parts of the body. Each consists of a bundle of tiny fibers no thicker than a human hair. But each fiber can support up to 1000 times its own weight. Yet research has shown that when a muscle isn't used very much, it weakens and grows smaller. (Just observe anyone who has had an arm or a leg isolated in a cast for several weeks or someone who has been sick in bed for several days.) And that goes for every muscle in the body.

Any muscle that's in good condition will feel better and work more efficiently than one that's not. Strong, well-toned muscles are important to the way each of us functions in our daily lives. They can help get rid of posture problems like rounded shoulders or a head that juts forward. They can virtually eliminate pot bellies and lower back pain. And they can improve blood circulation in the lower legs and other parts of the body. In addition, a good degree of muscular strength can make it easier to do the minor chores and other physical tasks each of us faces every day.

What is Flexibility?

Flexibility refers to the range of motion in a joint or sequence of joints, and it depends largely upon how supple and elastic the muscles are. A person with good flexibility is usually able to achieve a full range of movement in his or her joints. That means being able to touch your toes, do sit-ups, or generally move the parts of your body in any direction they are designed to go.

Good flexibility gives you freedom of movement. That can be essential in emergency situations, as when you have to quickly change body positions to avoid being hit by a falling object or oncoming vehicle. But flexibility is also essential to many of your normal daily activities. You may find that daily tasks such as tying your shoes, getting dressed, or bending over to pick up something have become painful experiences due to poor flexibility.

Most flexibility problems can be solved with the proper exercise. Muscles that are regularly stretched and moved throughout their full range of motion tend to remain elastic and supple. And joints, when exercised, tend to operate more smoothly.

Why Exercise is Essential

Whether you reach a normal level of fitness or not is pretty much a matter of choice. But you should realize that when a person chooses *not* to be fit, he or she is also choosing to become vulnerable to a whole range of physical problems.

By not being fit, for example, a person may be inviting chronic lower back pain caused by inadequate muscles and poor flexibility in the spine. Or accepting a state of constant fatigue. Or needlessly putting up with night after night of restless sleep.

As you exercise, all kinds of good things will begin happening in your body. Your heart will get stronger and your body's oxygen supply will improve. You'll have more stamina, endurance, and energy to perform your work and enjoy your free time. Muscle tone will increase and excess pounds will begin to disappear. You'll look better, feel better, be less susceptible to disease, and even sleep better once you're physically fit. You may even live longer, and you'll certainly enjoy your life more.

How to exercise

Once you've decided to begin exercising, you've got to choose a time during the day when you'll do your exercises. Physically, there's no reason why you must always exercise at the same time. But most people find that they do much better when they exercise at the same time on the designated exercise day. That way exercise becomes a part of the daily routine instead of something to be done on a catch-as-catch-can basis. And when exercise becomes a normal part of the day, it's much easier to stick with a regular program.

Another thing you've got to decide is how often to exercise. The programs in FULLY FIT IN 60 MINUTES A WEEK require that you exercise three times a week, 20 minutes each time. These workouts, when supplemented with your choice of a cardiovascular activity — walking, jogging, swimming or biking on alternate days — will leave you fully fit.

Begin the programs by deciding how many repetitions of each exercise you'll do. The number of repetitions is partly a physical decision, for there is naturally a limit to how many you *can* do at any given time. Still, it's a good idea to plan on starting slowly, by doing the fewest recommended repetitions and gradually working your way up. This is true even if you think you can do more at the beginning.

Physically, the most important form of preparation is the warm–up. This is a step that many people who don't know how to exercise often skip or overlook. You can't in FULLY FIT IN 60 MINUTES A WEEK — the warm–ups are part of the required 20-minute workouts. Skipping the warm–ups is an open invitation to a pulled muscle or some other injury.

In some ways your body is like a car on a winter morning. If you run it flat out right after starting it — before the engine has warmed up and before the oil has begun to circulate — you can stand a good chance of damaging it. Your body is the same way. When you warm up by doing some light stretching and flexibility exercises, you gradually raise your body temperature, increase your heart rate and respiration, and stretch out your muscles. Once you've done that, you can glide smoothly into more intense exercises and easily reach the level required for good conditioning.

Equally important is a warm down or cool down period after you've finished. When you exercise, your muscles create waste products that must be removed. During exercise this removal is no problem, since your blood is speeding around your body. But if you suddenly stop exercising, your circulation rate slows down, leaving some waste products "in the pipeline." It's these waste products that often cause a muscle to be stiff or sore. And while they will eventually be removed by the blood, the process will take much longer at a slower rate of circulation.

That's why it's a good idea to walk for a while, swinging your arms, and complete the recommended stretching exercises before you finish each session. Activities like these will keep your blood moving fast enough to remove most of the waste products created by your more intense exercise.

A cool or lukewarm shower is another good idea. If you take a hot shower, blood will rush to the surface of the skin to get rid of the heat, which may cause dizziness or other more serious problems. This rush of blood, combined with the blood flow caused by your recent exercise will raise your body temperature slightly. A cool or lukewarm shower will help your body get rid of excess heat.

Listed below are several reminders that will help make your exercise activities safe, beneficial, and enjoyable. You might want to give the list a quick once–over before you begin each exercise session until these suggestions become a habit.

Exercise Checklist —
The Do's and Don'ts of Fitness

1. Wear loose, non–binding clothing. This will make it easy to move and to avoid any restrictions of blood flow.

2. Warm up before doing the more vigorous exercises (this is also good advice for participating in sports or other recreational activities). Bending, stretching, running in place slowly, and other warm–up exercises are your best protections against injury.

Specific warm–up and flexibility exercises are given in this book.

3. Don't try to do too much too soon. Build up the intensity of your exercise gradually. Add one or two repetitions a day or every other day until you reach the desired number.

4. Always cool down after exercise. This will keep your circulation moving and help prevent muscle soreness.

5. Watch out for these warning signs:

    - fluttery, irregular pulse
    - unusual pain or pressure in the chest
    - pain or pressure in the arm or throat after exercise
    - dizziness
    - cold sweat
    - any abnormal body response

If any of these signs appear, stop exercising immediately and call a physician.

FULLY FIT IN 60 MINUTES A WEEK

MONDAY

WARM–UP: 5 minutes

Jog in place . . . . 1 min.–2 min.
Toe touches 15–30
Full arm circles. . . . . 20 each way
Body bends . . . . 10–20 each way
(5 4 count reps.)
Windmills. . . . . 5–10 4 count reps.

SHAPE–UP: 12 minutes

Sit–ups, crossarmed. . . . . 15–30 reps.
Pretzels. . . . . 5–7 reps. each side
Metronomes . . . . 6–20 sweeps (reps.)
Side leg raises. . . . . 10–30 each leg
Knee Push–ups or
    Push–ups. . . . . 10–30 reps.
Crossovers . . . . 5–10 4 count reps.
Backovers . . . . 5–7 reps.
Ball jumps. . . . . 20–120 jumps

COOL–DOWN: 3 minutes

Body bends . . . . 10–20 each way
Toe touches 15–30
Walk & deep breathing . . . . 60 sec.

Warm-up

**JOG OR RUN
IN PLACE**
1 min.–2 min.

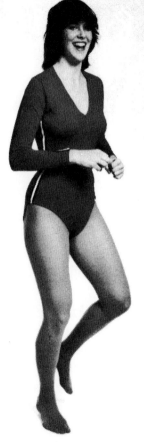

JOG OR RUN IN PLACE

Run slowly and softly, landing on each foot, toes first. Land gently on your toes or you will cause soreness of the calf muscles. The feet should be raised at least four inches off the floor. The benefit is improved cardiovascular and respiratory fitness; the heart becomes stronger and more efficient. Jogging also has a toning effect for the hips and thighs.

TOE
TOUCHES
15–30

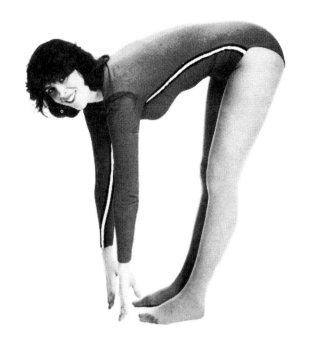

TOE TOUCHES

Starting Position: Stand erect with arms at sides.

The Movement: At the count of one, bend the trunk forward and down, flexing the knees slightly and touching the fingers to the ankles. At the count of two, return to the starting position.

The Benefit: This is a great stretcher. You can feel the gentle tugging from your calves through the derrière to the lower and upper back and arms.

Warm-up

FULL ARM
CIRCLES
20 each way

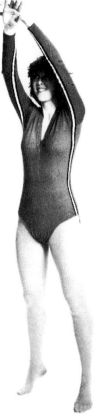

FULL ARM CIRCLES

Starting Position: Stand erect with the feet shoulder–width apart. Keep the arms at the side.

The Movement: Start slowly by bringing the arms upward and sideward, crossing overhead, and completing full arc in front of the body. As repetitions increase so should speed of swinging. Go slowly at first. Reverse the action.

The Benefit: This exercise will increase the muscle tone of the upper back and chest, and aid flexibility of the shoulder girdle.

**BODY
BENDS**
10–20 each
way (5 4–count
reps.)

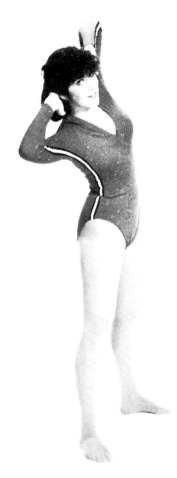

BODY BENDS

Starting Position: Stand erect with hands behind the neck, fingers interlaced. The feet should be shoulder–width apart.

The Movement: At the count of one, bend the trunk sideward to the left as far as possible, keeping the hands behind the neck. At the count of two, return to the starting position. Counts three and four repeat the exercise to the right.

The Benefit: This exercise works the waist and upper torso muscles; it will tone the flabby roll around the midsection.

Warm-up

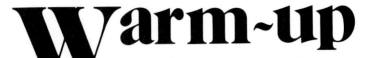

WINDMILLS
5–10   4–count
reps.

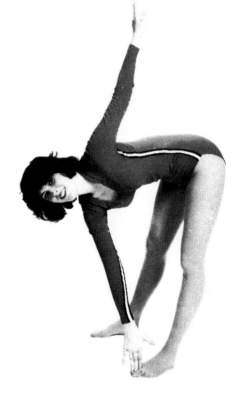

WINDMILLS

Starting Position: Stand erect with feet spread shoulder–width apart. Extend your hands sideward at shoulder level with palms down.

The Movement: At the count of one, bend and twist trunk from right to left, touching the right hand to left toe. At the count of two, return to the starting position. Counts three and four repeat the same action to the opposite side. Do this exercise with knees slightly flexed.

The Benefit: This is a good stretching exercise, especially for the muscles in the lower back, thighs and waistline.

Shape-up

SIT–UPS,
CROSS-
ARMED
15–30 reps.

SIT–UPS, CROSSARMED

Starting Position: Lie on your back with legs bent and arms crossed, hands grasping the opposite shoulders.

The Movement: At the count of one, roll up to a sitting position. Exhale as you sit as far forward as possible before returning to the starting position at the count of two.

The Benefit: This exercise increases the abdominal muscle tone.

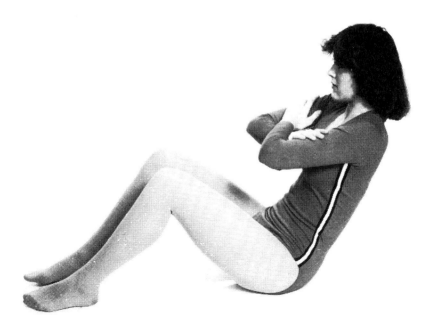

Shape-up

PRETZELS

PRETZELS
5–7 reps. each side

Starting Position: Sit on the floor with your left leg straight out, then cross your right leg over the left one, placing your right foot flat on the floor. With your left hand, reach right in front of you and toward your right hip. Place your right hand on the floor directly behind you.

The Movement: Sitting up very straight, slowly turn your head toward the right and look over your right shoulder. Hold for 10 counts. Repeat to the opposite side.

The Benefit: This exercise gently stretches the back muscles.

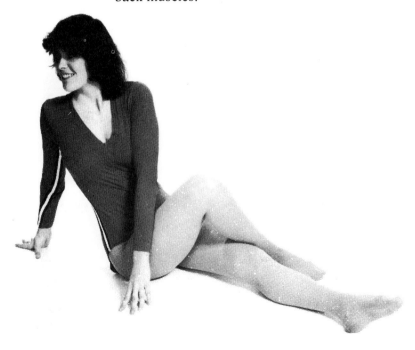

METRO-
NOMES
6–20 sweeps
(reps.)

METRONOMES

Starting Position: Lying flat on your back, extend arms out to each side and raise both legs straight up in the air together.

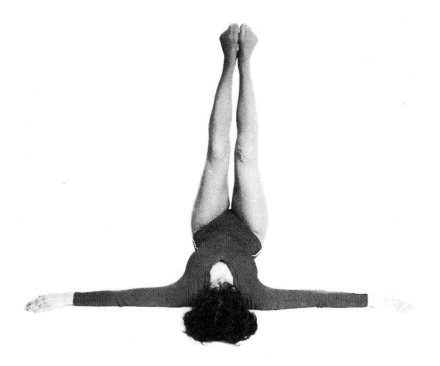

Shape-up

The Movement: Swing legs to one side, almost to floor (but not touching!). Swing legs over to the other side, then back to the starting position. One side–to–side sweep equals a repetition.

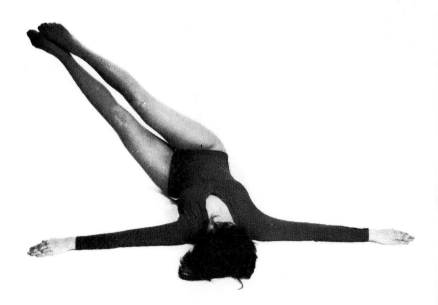

The Benefit: This exercise is very good for strengthening your lower back, waist, hips and abdominal muscles, and reducing "love handles."

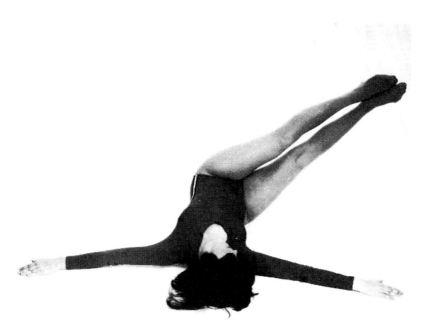

Shape-up

SIDE LEG RAISES

Starting Position: Lie on your right side with your head resting on the right hand, right elbow resting on the floor.

The Movement: At the count of one, lift the left leg as high as possible. On the count of two, lower the leg to the starting position. Then reverse the position and repeat the exercise on the other side.

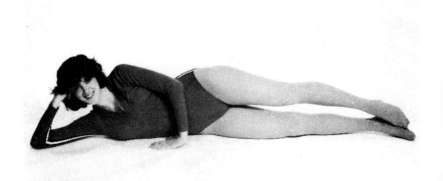

The Benefit: This exercise brings into play the lateral muscles of the legs and hips. It also serves to slim the waistline by toning the sides of the torso.

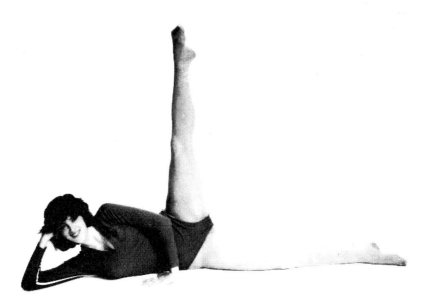

Shape~up

KNEE PUSH–UPS OR PUSH–UPS*

Starting Position: Lie on the floor face down, legs together and knees bent with the feet raised off the floor. The hands should be placed directly under the shoulders with the palms down and fingers pointed straight ahead.

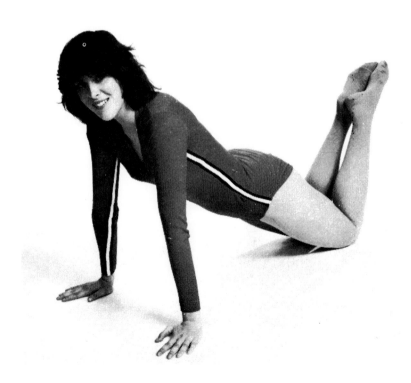

The Movement: At the count of one, push the upper body off the floor until the arms are fully extended and the body is straight from the head to the knees. There should not be a sag in the middle. At count two, return to the starting position.

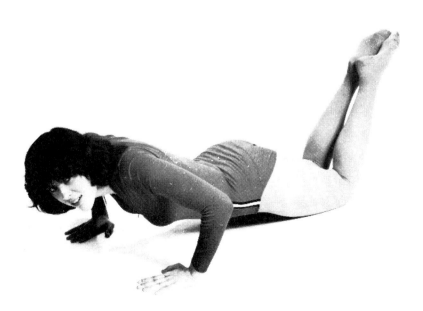

Shape-up

The Benefit: This exercise will strengthen the back of the arms and the shoulder girdle, and increase the muscular tone of the muscles that support the bust.

*Starting position is balanced on toes.

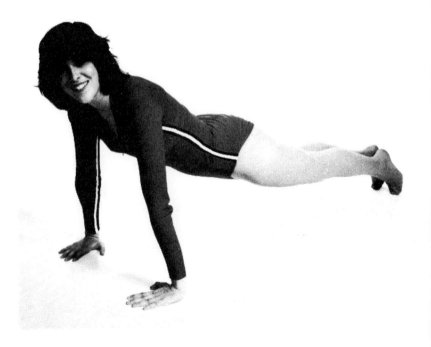

CROSSOVERS

Starting Position: Lie on back, legs together, arms extended sideward, palms down.

The Movement: At the count of one, raise the left leg to vertical position and lower across body to floor in attempt to touch fingertips of right hand. At count two, return to the starting position. Counts three and four repeat the action to the opposite side.

The Benefit: Stretches the lower back, upper leg and waist muscles; strengthens the abdominals.

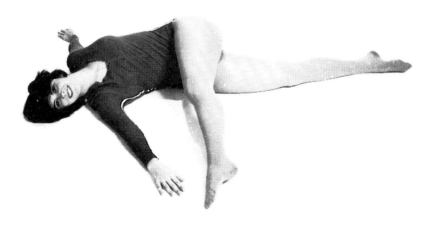

Shape~up

BACKOVERS
5–7 reps.

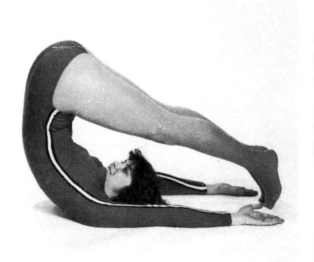

BACKOVERS

Starting Position: Lie on the floor with arms extended over your head.

The Movement: While exhaling, bring your legs over your head and as close to the floor as possible. Hold this position for 5 counts and, while inhaling, return to starting position.

The Benefit: This exercise stretches the back muscles and strengthens abdominal muscles.

BALL JUMPS
20–120 jumps

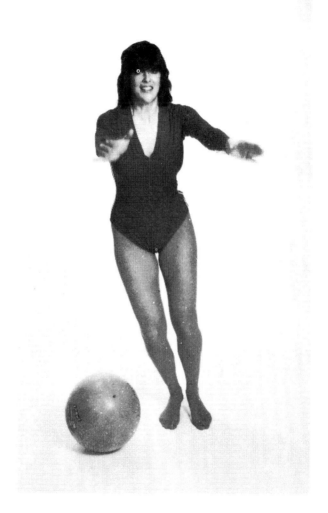

BALL JUMPS

Starting Position: Stand alongside a plastic or rubber ball approximately 16" in diameter with feet together.

Shape~up

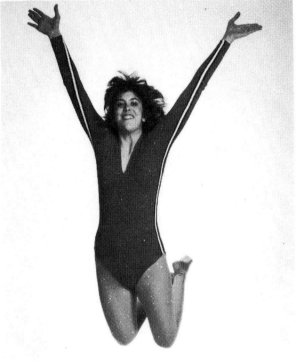

The Movement: Jump sideways over the ball. Repeat rapidly, jumping from one side of the ball to the other.

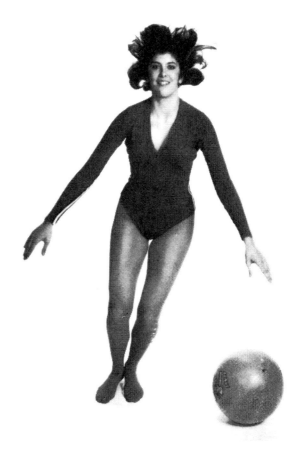

The Benefit: This one really gets the blood pumping, is great for your circulatory system, and puts your coordination to the test.

Cool~down

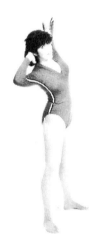

BODY BENDS: 10–20 each way

TOE TOUCHES: 15–30

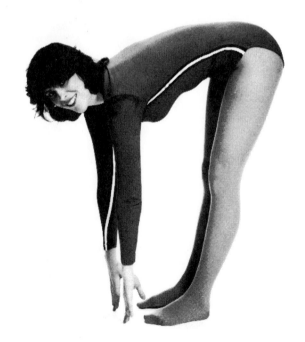

WALK & DEEP BREATHING: 60 sec.

WEDNESDAY

WARM–UP: 5 minutes

Jog in place . . . . 1 min.–2 min.
Side bends . . . . 10–20 each way
Toe touches 15–30
Full arm circles . . . . 20 each way
Windmills . . . . 5–10 4 count reps.

SHAPE–UP: 12 minutes

Leg circles . . . . 10–30 reps. each leg/3 sets
Knee Push–ups or
    Push–ups . . . . 10–30 reps.
Sitting leg kicks . . . . 20–40 reps./4 sets
Alternate leg knee pulls 5–7
Sit–ups, crossarmed . . . . 15–30 reps.
Lateral arm raises . . . . . . 10–30 each arm/2 sets
Scrunch/Screams . . . . 6 reps./5 sec. each
Bust builders . . . . 30 reps./5 sets

COOL–DOWN: 3 minutes

Side bends . . . . 10–20 each way
Toe touches 15–30
Walk & deep breathing . . . . 60 sec.

Warm-up

SIDE BENDS
10–20 each way

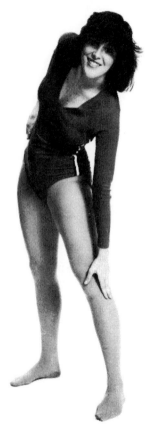

SIDE BENDS

Starting Position: Stand upright with your hands at your sides and your feet spread to shoulder width.

The Movement: Bend the trunk to the right until resistance is felt, then return to upright position. Then bend to the left and repeat.

The Benefit: This is an excellent stretching exercise for the hips and waist.

Shape~up

LEG
CIRCLES
10–30 reps.
each leg/
3 sets

LEG CIRCLES

Starting Position: Assume a comfortable position on your hands and knees, head up.

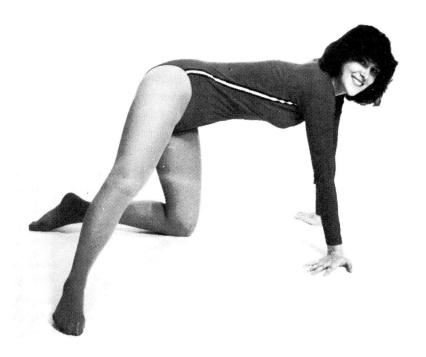

Shape-up

The Movement: Thrust one leg out to the side and rotate forward and clockwise in wide circles. Complete the recommended number of circles and resume the starting position. Repeat the exercise with the other leg.

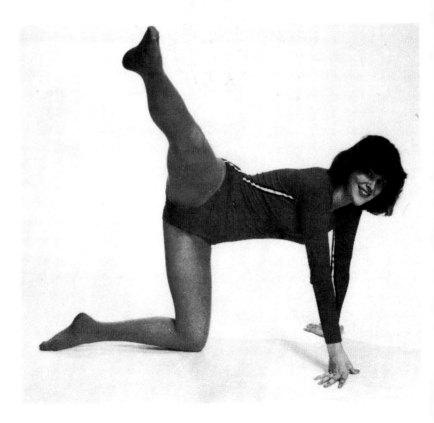

The Benefit: This exercise is very good for firming your thighs, waist and derrière.

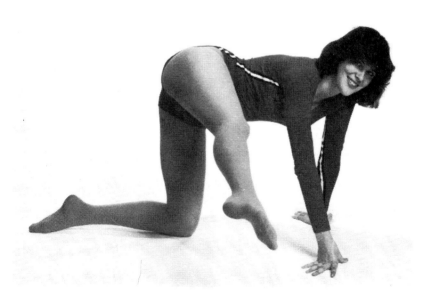

Shape~up

**SITTING
LEG KICKS**
20–40 reps.
4 sets

SITTING LEG KICKS

Starting Position: Sit with legs extended, hands flat on the floor, fingers pointing sideward. Lean backward, bend the knees, and lift the feet off the floor.

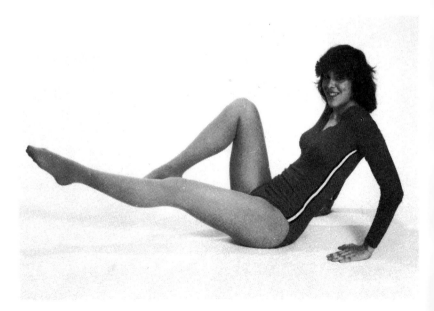

The Movement: Alternately straighten one leg while the other is flexed.

The Benefit: These kicks tone the abdominal and thigh muscles.

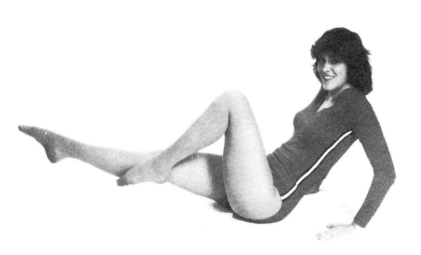

Shape-up

ALTERNATE LEG KNEE PULLS

Starting Position: Lie on your back with both legs extended, arms at your sides.

The Movement: Pull one leg up to your chest, grasp leg with both arms and hold for a 5 count. Repeat this exercise with the other leg.

The Benefit: This exercise stretches and firms thigh muscles and tones the derrière and hips.

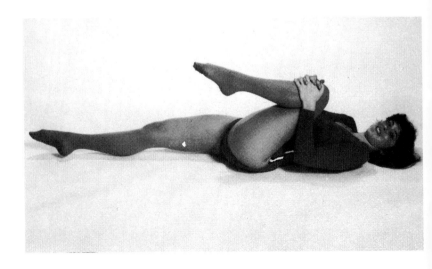

**LATERAL
ARM
RAISES**
10–30 each
arm 2 sets

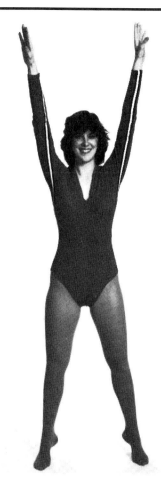

LATERAL ARM RAISES

Starting Position: Stand erect, feet together, with your arms at your sides.

The Movement: Taking a slow, deep breath, lift arms sideward and upward at count one and raise onto toes slightly. At count two, exhale slowly while returning to starting position.

The Benefit: This exercise conditions the waist, upper arms and shoulders.

Shape~up

**SCRUNCH/
SCREAMS**
6 reps./5 sec.
each

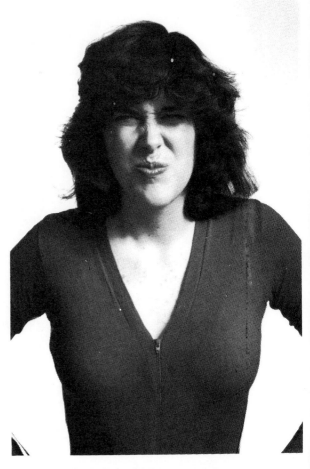

SCRUNCH/SCREAMS

Starting Position: Sit or stand erect with hands at your waist.

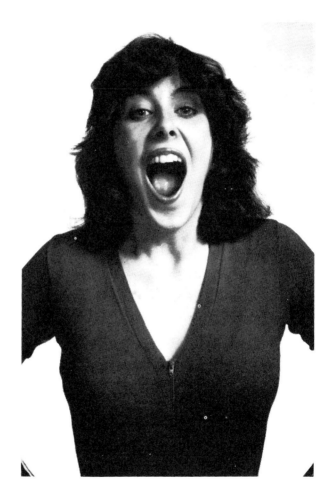

The Movement: Concentrate on making your face as small as possible, and then make it as large as possible, as in screaming. Hold each expression for five seconds.

The Benefit: This exercise tones the facial muscles.

Shape ~ up

**BUST
BUILDERS**
30 reps./5 sets

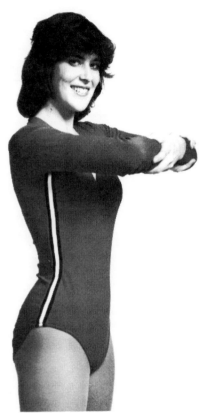

BUST BUILDERS

Starting Position: From a standing or sitting position, grasp both forearms with opposite hands. Keep arms approximately four inches from the body, chest high.

The Movement: Rapidly and vigorously push both arms together. Rest and then repeat action.

Cool~down

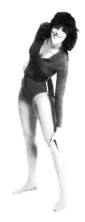

SIDE BENDS: 10–20 each way

TOE TOUCHES 15–30

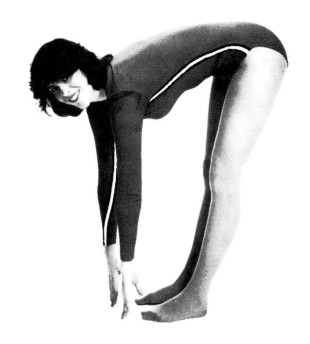

WALK & DEEP BREATHING: 60 sec.

FRIDAY

WARM–UP: 5 minutes
Jog in place . . . . 1 min.–2 min.
Windmills. . . . . 5–10 4 count reps.
Body bends . . . . 10–20 each way
(5 4 count reps.)
Full arm circles. . . . . 20 each way
Toe touches 15–30

SHAPE–UP: 12 minutes
Stair stretches . . . . 5 reps.
Scrunch/Screams . . . . 6 reps.–5 secs. each
Sit–ups, crossarmed 15–30
Bust builders . . . . 30 reps./5 sets
Lateral arm raises with
dumbell. . . . . 10–30 each arm/2 sets
Knee Push–ups or
Push–ups. 10–30 reps.
Crossovers . . . . 5–10 4 count reps./2 sets
Double leg knee pulls 5–7

COOL–DOWN: 3 minutes
Body bends . . . . 10–20 each way
Toe touches 15–30
Walk & deep breathing . . . . 60 sec.

Shape~up

**STAIR
STRETCHES**
5 reps.

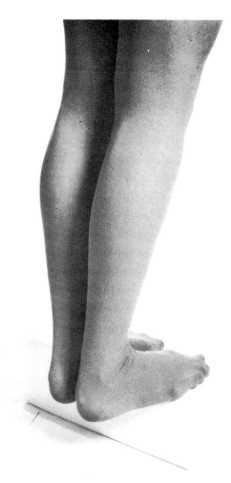

STAIR STRETCHES

Starting Position: Stand on the edge of a step or curb with your heels
halfway off.

Shape-up

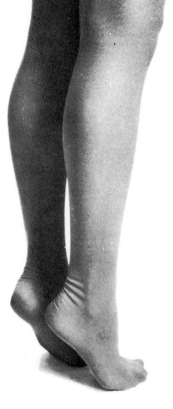

The Movement: Rise up on your toes and hold this position for a count of ten. Next, press your heels down below the step and hold again for a count of ten; or for maximum benefit, press down one foot at a time.

The Benefit: This exercise safely stretches the Achilles' tendon, which attaches the calf muscle to your heel.

DOUBLE
LEG KNEE PULLS

Starting Position: Lie on your back with both legs extended, arms at your sides.

The Movement: Pull both legs to your chest, lock arms around legs, pulling the buttocks slightly off the floor, and hold for 20–25 counts.

The Benefit: This tones the hips, derrière, and thighs.

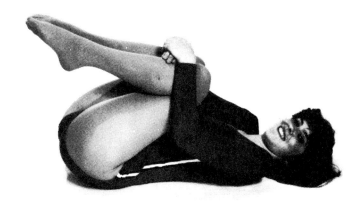

Cool~down

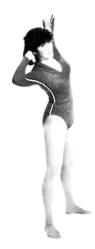

BODY BENDS: 10–20 each way

TOE TOUCHES: 15–30

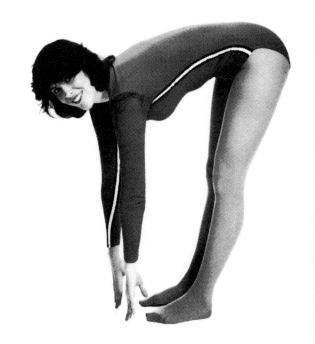

WALK & DEEP BREATHING: 60 sec.

Oooh...But I'm So Sore, Help!

Many people think that if you don't feel stiff and sore after an exercise session, you haven't worked hard enough. Not true. Proper exercising is started slowly and intensified over a period of time. Overwork and too much enthusiasm in the beginning only result in muscle soreness and poor performance on the following days. So take it slow and you'll minimize muscle discomfort.

The descriptions that follow are intended to serve as a guide for identifying the nature of the discomfort and relieving it through proven first aid treatment. Lesser injuries can be treated by following these simple directions. More serious injuries or those that result in extreme loss of motion of the muscles and joints should be examined by a doctor.

General Muscle Soreness

This is a feeling of stiffness and aching in the muscles, usually experienced twelve to twenty–four hours after a workout. This condition occurs in almost everyone who works out, even in trained athletes. It always follows the first workout of an inactive person.

When exercise is resumed the day after soreness sets in, it will cause pain; this usually disappears after two to three minutes of activity. When the exercising is ended, however, the soreness reappears to a lesser degree.

Soreness can be minimized by a progressive series of exercises calling for harder workouts after periods of milder ones, and by adequate tapering off of the exercise program each day. The workouts in FULLY FIT IN 60 MINUTES A WEEK are so designed.

One of the by–products of muscle exercising is lactic acid. If it is not removed from the cells by tapering off methods, muscle soreness results. If a regular program of exercise is maintained for at least two weeks, this type of soreness will gradually disappear. It usually takes this long for the skeletal–muscular system to become accustomed to the workout.

Muscle Cramps

These are prolonged, painful contractions of one or more muscles. They are most often experienced in the legs or feet. Flexing and massage will help alleviate the condition and restore the muscle to the near–normal state of tension.

An inadequate amount of warm–ups is the most prevalent cause of cramps. If cramps occur on a regular basis, a physician should be consulted.

Sprains

A sprain involves the twisting of a joint, with subsequent tearing and stretching of the ligaments supporting the joint. A severe sprain often involves injury to the surrounding nerves and muscles.

The treatment is ice application, rest, and elevation of the injured area followed by an x–ray to determine the extent of the injury. Heat is not applied to a sprain for at least thirty–six hours after the injury. A sprain should always be looked at by a doctor for complete diagnosis and treatment.

Strains

A strain involves the actual tearing of a muscle fiber. The seriousness of the injury depends on the amount of fibers involved in the tear.

This overstretching of the muscle fibers is often the result of a maximum effort without proper warm–up. To remember how your muscles react when properly warmed up, consider the modest analogy between muscle fibers and taffy. After having been kneaded and stretched a piece of taffy is capable of maximum tensions and twisting without tearing. Try the twisting and pulling when it is cold, and it will break. Your muscles respond the same way; extend them when they are cold, and they will tear and rupture.

Athletes commonly refer to strains as "pulled muscles" or "muscle pulls." When use of the strained, or "pulled" muscle is required, there is severe discomfort and pain. The treatment is the immediate application of ice to reduce the swelling and capillary bleeding. After thirty-six hours heat may be applied. When possible the injury should be protected against further injury by adhesive taping. Immediate resumption of activity is not recommended, as the weaker fibrous scar tissue, which is replacing the torn muscle, is prone to further injury.

Contusions

A contusion is the result of a blow to some portion of the body causing tissue tearing and hemorrhaging. The injured area appears red and swollen; the muscle is usually immobilized after a short time. Contusions are common to the quadriceps (or thighs) and are more commonly known as "charley horses."

The immediate treatment of any contusion should be to pack it with ice. After thirty–six hours heat should be applied; this will help to reduce the swelling. An examination by a doctor is recommended in order to determine the extent of deep tissue damage.